A. Newman

Comparison of the Mortality from Disease in Armies

With that of Men of Military Ages in Civil Life Showing the Groups of

Diseases Chiefly Concerned in Causing the Excess of Mortality in Armies

A. Newman

Comparison of the Mortality from Disease in Armies
*With that of Men of Military Ages in Civil Life Showing the Groups of Diseases
Chiefly Concerned in Causing the Excess of Mortality in Armies*

ISBN/EAN: 9783337427900

Printed in Europe, USA, Canada, Australia, Japan

Cover: Foto ©Suzi / pixelio.de

More available books at **www.hansebooks.com**

COMPARISON

OF THE

MORTALITY FROM DISEASE IN ARMIES,

WITH THAT OF

Men of Military Ages = Civil Life

SHOWING THE

GROUPS OF DISEASES CHIEFLY CONCERNED IN CAUSING
THE EXCESS OF MORTALITY IN ARMIES.

By A. NEWMAN, M. D., LAWRENCE, KANSAS.

LEAVENWORTH :
TIMES AND CONSERVATIVE PRINTING HOUSE, 13 & 15 SHAWNEE STREET.
1869.

COMPARISON

OF THE

MORTALITY FROM DISEASE IN ARMIES,

WITH THAT OF

Men of Military Ages : Civil Life

SHOWING THE

GROUPS OF DISEASES CHIEFLY CONCERNED IN CAUSING
THE EXCESS OF MORTALITY IN ARMIES.

By A. NEWMAN, M. D., LAWRENCE, KANSAS.

LEAVENWORTH:
TIMES AND CONSERVATIVE PRINTING HOUSE, 13 & 15 SHAWNEE STREET.
1869.

A COMPARISON OF THE MORTALITY FROM DISEASE IN ARMIES, WITH THAT OF MEN OF MILITARY AGES IN CIVIL LIFE, SHOWING THE GROUPS OF DISEASES CHIEFLY CONCERNED IN CAUSING THE EXCESS OF MORTALITY IN ARMIES.

When we compare the mortality from disease in armies, with that of men of military ages in civil life, we find a striking difference in favor of civil life. As soldiers are ordinarily subjected to a rigid examination before enlistment, which causes the exclusion, not only of all who are subjects of disease, but also of all of feeble constitutions, we might reasonably expect that, all other things being equal, the mortality from disease in armies would be considerably below that of men of military ages in civil life. And even when no preliminary examination is had, as was the case in many of our volunteer regiments organized during the early part of the war, since comparatively few who did not consider themselves possessed of ordinary vigor and powers of endurance would be likely to volunteer, the vital standard of the army would still be considerably above that of men of military ages in civil life as a whole; and under equally favorable circumstances, therefore, it would be reasonable to expect that the mortality from disease in armies would be less than in civil life.

The total number of deaths from disease during the year ending June 1st, 1860, in a male population between the ages of fifteen and fifty, of 8,068,595, was, according to the last United States Census, 50,961, or about 6.3 per 1000 of population between the ages of fifteen and fifty. It would be unreasonable to assume, however, that this represents the total mortality occurring during the year in men of military ages in the United States. Such statistics are necessarily much less complete in civil life than in armies. Many deaths would be likely to occur during the year, of which the census officers would get no information.

In estimating the total mortality therefore, of men of military ages in civil life, the incompleteness of mortality returns must be considered. It is not probable, however, that if the whole number of deaths had been reported, it would have raised the mortality of men of military ages above 10 per 1000. This would be assuming that but little over three-fifths of the actual number of deaths was reported, which is certainly a very ample allowance for the presumed incompleteness of the census returns. This corresponds also with the estimated mortality from disease of men of military ages in Europe. Now when we inquire respecting the annual mortality of armies from disease, we find that instead of being less than 10 per 1000 of mean strength, as we might expect, if no new causes of disease were brought into action, it has, invariably, in all military campaigns, been many times greater. At Walcheren in 1809, the British Army lost 332 per 1000 by disease. In Burmah the mortality from disease reached 450 per 1000. In the British Crimean Army, the mortality from disease was 232 per 1000; and in the French Crimean Army nearly or quite 300 per 1000 of mean strength. In our own armies, in the Mexican war, the annual mortality from disease was 103.8, and in the last war, during the first year, 48.7, and during the second year 65.2. These figures, strikingly small as they are, when compared with the mortality of any large army in any previous military campaign, are evidently greatly in excess of the ordinary mortality of men of military ages in civil life. What were the causes which contributed most to make the mortality from disease in our armies, composed of the most vigorous and robust of our citizens, almost five times as great during the first year of the war, and over six and a half times as great during the second year, as that of men of the same ages in civil life? The fact that our volunteer army was composed largely of men of decided intelligence and morality, and of respectable social standing, makes the result of a comparison of the mortality statistics of the armies of the United States, and of the male citizens of the United States, of military ages, exceedingly trustworthy and reliable. For the purpose of comparison with the mortality statistics of our armies, the territory of the United States has been divided into three regions, namely: the Atlantic region; comprising the six New England States, New York, New Jersey, Pennsylvania, Delaware, Maryland, the District of Columbia, Virginia, North and South Carolina, Georgia, Florida and Alabama, (this includes districts 1, 3, 5 and 7 of the census report, and embraces all the territory of the United States, east of the Appalachian range of mountains, sometimes called the Atlantic slope); the Central Region, comprising the states of Michigan, Wisconsin, Minnesota, Nebraska, Ohio, Indiana, Illinois, Iowa, Kansas, Kentucky, Tennessee, Missouri Mississippi, Louisiana, Arkansas and Texas, and constituting districts 2, 4, 6 and 8 of the census report; (this region includes the territory of the United States between the Appalachian and Rocky Mountain ranges and embraces all the rich alluvial bottoms of the Mississippi River and its tributaries); and the Pacific region, comprising the states of Oregon and California and the territories of Dakota, New Mexico, Utah and Washington, and embracing the territory west of the Rocky Mountains, (this region corresponds with district 9 of the census report). By reason of the presumed incompleteness of the mortality returns the ratios of deaths per 1000 of population, as shown in the following tables, is undoubtedly too low; but as the deaths not reported, would be likely to be distributed among the several diseases and classes of diseases, in about the same proportions as those reported the ratio of reported deaths, from any disease or class of diseases to the total number of reported deaths, may be safely assumed as exhibiting very correctly the relative mortality of each of the several diseases and classes of diseases, as compared with each other. In the construction of these tables, I have followed the classification used in the reports of sick and wounded in the army, that the comparison may be more easy and intelligible. At the same time, I think it is to be regretted that the name "zymotic," should have been so universally adopted, and applied to a large number of diseases exceedingly diverse in nature, and produced by diverse causes, some of which, at least have no relation whatever with others. This name is based upon an hypothesis wholly unsupported by facts, and which, there is good reason to believe, is wholly untrue. It has now however, beccme so generally interwoven in the nomenclature of disease, that it must long remain as a monument of the error in which it originated.

In respect to the reliability of mortality statistics generally, it is evident that if our inquiries are directed only to determining the relative prevalence, or fatality of whole classes or orders of diseases, our conclusions will be more reliable and trustworthy than if we extend our inquiries to the prevalence and fatality of individual diseases. In the reports of sick and wounded in our armies, for example, which are undoubtedly more correct, as well as more complete, than those obtained in civil life, a certain number of cases of fever are reported as typhus, a certain number as typhoid, a certain number as typho-malarial, and a certain number as remittent. It would, however, be unreasonable to assume that the diagnosis was so correctly made in all these cases, that these reports furnish us sufficient data from which to determine the relative prevalence and fatality of each of these species of fever. Undoubtedly, precisely, similar cases were reported by some surgeons under one of these heads, and by other surgeons under different heads. But if, instead of inquiring respecting the prevalence and fatality of individual diseases, the resemblances of which would cause them often to be confounded, we limit our inquiries to the prevalence and fatality of classes, or orders of diseases, separated from each other by well marked lines and differences, this source of error will, to a great extent, disappear.

TABLE NO. 1.

Deaths of Male Citizens of the United States between the ages of fifteen and fifty, during the year ending June 1st, 1860, from the Several Classes of Diseases, with the Ratio of such Deaths per 1000 of Population of Corresponding Ages, and, also, per 1000 of deaths from all Diseases by Regions.

CLASSES.	ATLANTIC REGION.			CENTRAL REGION.			PACIFIC REGION.			TOTAL.		
	DEATHS.	Ratio per 1000 of Male population betwen the ages of 15 and 50.	Ratio per 1000 of deaths of males between the ages of 15 and 50, from all diseases.	DEATHS.	Ratio per 1000 of male population between the ages of 15 and 50.	Ratio per 1000 of deaths of males between the ages of 15 and 50, from all diseases.	DEATHS.	Ratio per 1000 of male population between the ages of 15 and 50.	Ratio per 1000 of deaths of males between the ages of 15 and 50, from all diseases.	DEATHS.	Ratio per 1000 of male population between the ages of 15 and 50.	Ratio per 1000 of deaths of males between the ages of 15 and 50, from all diseases.
1. Zymotic Diseases, ...	5,680	1.35	216.11	7,210	2.02	306.93	271	.90	228.30	13,161	1.63	258.26
2. Constitutional Diseases,....	10,577	2.52	402.42	6,664	1.87	283.68	426	1.42	358.89	17,667	2.19	346.68
3. Parasitic Diseases,.........	6	.001	.23	6	.001	.25	2	.007	1.69	14	.02	.28
4. Local Diseases,......	7,744	1.85	294.64	7,852	2.20	334.26	352	1.17	296.55	15,948	1.98	312.94
5. Unclassified Diseases,....	2,276	.54	86.60	1,759	.49	74.88	136	.45	114.57	4,171	.52	81.84
Total,..........	26,283	6.26	1000.00	23,491	6.58	1000.00	1,187	3.95	1000.00	50,961	6.34	1000.00

This table shows, if the statistics from which it is constructed are reliable, that in the whole United States, more deaths are produced in men of military ages by the constitutional diseases than by any other class; the mortality from this class being 347 of every 1000 deaths. Next to this class stand local diseases, the mortality from which was 313 of every 1000 deaths; while the so-called zymotic diseases represent a mortality of 258 of every 1000 deaths, or a little over one fourth of the whole. If we compare the mortality in the different regions, we find that in the Atlantic and Pacific Regions, the constitutional diseases are decidedly more fatal than any other class, causing 359 deaths of every 1000 in the Pacific Region, and 402 of every 1000 in the Atlantic Region. We find here, also, that the local diseases stand next, their proportional fatality scarcely differing in the two regions, being 295 of every 1000 in the Atlantic Region, and 297 of every 1000 in the Pacific Region; while the proportional mortality from the zymotic diseases is but 216 of every 1000 in the Atlantic Region, and 228 of every 1000 in the Pacific Region, ranging between one fifth and one fourth of the total mortality. In the Central Region, however, we find these proportions considerably changed, and the constitutional diseases decidedly the least fatal of the three important classes, representing a mortality of but 284 of every 1000 deaths, while local diseases, here the most fatal class, cause 334 of every 1000 deaths, or one third of the whole; and zymotic diseases 307 of every 1000. There are two facts which serve to explain these differences: 1st, in a considerable portion of the territory included in the Central Region, the mortality from consumption, is greatly below the average in the whole United States, while in the whole northern portion of the Atlantic Region, and especially in the New England States, the mortality from this disease is very great; 2nd, the Central Region includes all the rich alluvial bottoms of the Mississippi River and its tributaries, and we might therefore reasonably expect, that the miasmatic diseases especially, would be more prevalent and fatal in this region, than in either of the other two; and we accordingly find that the smaller relative mortality from the constitutional diseases in this region, depends both upon an absolutely smaller mortality from this class of diseases in this region, than in the other regions, and, also upon an absolutely larger mortality from both the zymotic and local diseases. The several classes of diseases therefore, arranged in the order of their relative mortality in men of military ages in civil life, if we speak of the whole United States, or of either the Atlantic or Pacific Region, will stand; 1st, constitutional diseases; 2nd, local diseases; 3rd, zymotic diseases. But if we speak of the Central Region alone, they will stand; 1st, local diseases; 2nd, zymotic diseases; 3rd, constitutional diseases. Let us compare these results with the mortality in our armies, serving in corresponding regions of territory.

2

TABLE NO. 2.

Deaths in the Armies of the United States during the year ending June 30th, 1862, from the Several Classes of Diseases, with the Ratio of such Deaths per 1000 of Mean Strength, and also per 1000 of Deaths from all Diseases, by Regions.

CLASSES.	ATLANTIC REGION.			CENTRAL REGION.			PACIFIC REGION.			TOTAL.		
	DEATHS.	Ratio per 1000 of mean strength.	Ratio per 1000 of deaths from all diseases.	DEATHS.	Ratio per 1000 of mean strength.	Ratio per 1000 of deaths from all diseases.	DEATHS.	Ratio per 1000 of mean strength.	Ratio per 1000 of deaths from all diseases.	DEATHS.	Ratio per 1000 of mean strength.	Ratio per 1000 of deaths from all diseases.
1. Zymotic Diseases,	4,032	22.08	677.19	5,269	51.83	646.34	32	4.78	415.58	9,333	32.08	658.04
2. Constitutional Diseases,	285	1.56	47.87	367	3.61	45.02	14	2.09	181.82	666	2.29	46.96
3. Parasitic Diseases,												
4. Local Diseases,	1,375	7.53	230.94	2,341	23.03	287.17	26	3.88	337.65	3,742	12.86	263.84
5. Unclassified Diseases,	262	1.43	44.00	175	1.72	21.47	5	.75	64.94	442	1.52	31.16
Total,	5,954	32.60	1000.00	8,152	80.19	1000.00	77	11.50	1000.00	14,183	48.75	1000.00

TABLE NO. 3.

Deaths in the Armies of the United States during the Year ending June 30th, 1863, from the Several Classes of Diseases, with the Ratio of such Deaths per 1000 of Mean Strength, and also per 1000 of Deaths from all Diseases, by Regions.

CLASSES.	ATLANTIC REGION.			CENTRAL REGION.			PACIFIC REGION.			TOTAL.		
	DEATHS.	Ratio per 1000 of mean strength.	Ratio per 1000 of deaths from all diseases.	DEATHS.	Ratio per 1000 of mean strength.	Ratio per 1000 of deaths from all diseases.	DEATHS.	Ratio per 1000 of mean strength.	Ratio per 1000 of deaths from all diseases.	DEATHS.	Ratio per 1000 of mean stren h.	Ratio per 1000 of deaths from all diseases.
1. Zymotic Diseases,	9,529	30.59	738.85	20.158	62.16	694.15	23	2.64	315.07	29,710	46.10	707.22
2. Constitutional Diseases,	812	2.61	62.96	1,736	5.35	59.78	8	.92	109.59	2,556	3.97	60.84
3. Parasitic Diseases,	1	.003	.08							1	.002	.02
4. Local Diseases,	2,555	8.20	198.11	7,146	22.04	246.07	42	4.82	575.34	9,743	15.12	231.92
Total,	12,897	41.40	1000.00	29,040	89.55	1000.00	73	8.38	1000.00	42,010	65.19	1000.00

The first thing that strikes us upon examining these tables, is the great relative mortality from the zymotic diseases. In the Atlantic Region, we see that instead of causing but little over one fifth of the total mortality from disease as in civil life, this class of diseases caused two thirds of all the deaths from disease in the armies serving in this region during the first year of the war, and almost three fourths of the whole, during the second year. In the Central Region, although this relative excess is somewhat less, the relative mortality is still considerably over twice as great as in the same region in civil life. In the Pacific Region, in which the total mortality from disease, if we take the two years together, almost exactly corresponds with the estimated mortality of men of military ages in civil life, we still find that the relative mortality from this class of diseases is greatly in excess of that in civil life, being, during the first year of the war 416, and during the second year 315 of every 1000 deaths, instead of 228 per 1000 as in civil life.

The small relative mortality from the constitutional diseases is scarcely less striking. We find that while in the Atlantic Region, this class of diseases caused 402 of every 1000 deaths in civil life, in the armies serving in the same region it caused but 48 of every 1000 deaths during the first year, and 63 of every 1000 during the second year; and in the Central Region instead of 284 per 1000 as in civil life, but 45 during the first year and 60 during the second, the relative mortality from this class of diseases being almost the same in both these regions. In the Pacific Region, the relative mortality from this class of diseases is considerably greater, but it is still but little over half as great as that produced by the same class of diseases in the same region in civil life; and if we compare the mortality of the whole army with that of men of military ages in the whole United States, we find that, while of every 1000 deaths from disease in civil life, the constitutional diseases caused 347, in the whole army during the first year they caused but 47, and during the second year but 61 of every 1000. That this class of diseases should be less prevalent and fatal in an army, from which all affected with organic diseases, or possessing evident predisposition to such diseases, are excluded, than in civil life, is precisely what we ought to expect. The absolute mortality from this class of diseases however, is not so small as might, at first, be inferred from the small relative mortality shown to be produced by it, by this mode of comparison. The great excess of deaths from zymotic diseases would make the relative mortality from other classes smaller than in civil life even if they bore the same ratio to the whole number of living. But, in respect to this class of diseases, we find, that while in civil life, with returns which are known to be very incomplete, we have reported in the whole United States 2.19 deaths per 1000 of the population, in the whole army during the first year, with every death reported, there was but 2.29 per 1000 of mean strength

The ratio of deaths from this class of diseases per 1000 of mean strength, during the first year of the war, was probably but little over half as great as in civil life. During the second year, however, the mortality from this class of diseases, reached almost four per 1000 of mean strength, and probably approximated very closely to that in civil life. We find also, in respect to the mortality from local diseases, that it is relatively larger in civil life than in our army, causing in civil life 313 of every 1000 deaths, against 264 of every 1000 in the army during the first year, and 232 of every 1000 during the second year. A further examination, however, will show that the relatively smaller mortality from this class of diseases in the army, than in civil life, is due chiefly to the enormous increase in the mortality from the zymotic diseases in the army; and that the proportional mortality from local diseases, is less in the army than in civil life, only because it has not been so largely increased by the influences and exposures to which soldiers are subjected, as the mortality from the zymotic diseases has been. A comparison however, of the ratios of deaths per 1000 of mean strength or population, clearly shows that there is a much greater absolute mortality from the local diseases in the army than in civil life. We see from the first table, that the mortality from this class of diseases is greatest in the Central Region, and least in the Pacific Region, and that the ratio of reported deaths to population in the whole United States is about two per 1000. From table No. 2, we see that the mortality from this class of diseases in the army, serving in the Pacific Region, and which shared few of the exposures or hardships incident to a state of active warfare, scarcely reached four per 1000 of mean strength. As the total mortality of the army in this region, closely approximates to the estimated mortality of men of military ages in civil life, it is, I think, safe to assume that in men of military ages in civil life, the mortality from this class of diseases does not ordinarily exceed four per 1000 of living. But we find that in the army, the mortality from this class of diseases, was during the first year of the war, 7.5 per 1000 of mean strength in the Atlantic Region, and 23 per 1000 of mean strength in the Central Region; and in the whole army 12.8 per 1000. During the second year of the war, the mortality, from this class of diseases in the whole army became augmented to 15 per 1000 of mean strength, the increase being confined to the Pacific and Atlantic Regions. It would seem, therefore, that the mortality from local diseases in our army, was over three times as great during the first year of the war, and almost four times as great during the second year, as in men of military ages in civil life. The relative mortality from the several classes of diseases in our armies, was therefore, exactly the reverse of that in civil life; and arranged in the order of their relative fatality in the army, they stand; 1st, zymotic diseases; 2d, local diseases; 3d, constitutional diseases. And we find further that this change in the order of their relative importance has been brought about; 1st, by an enormous increase in the mortality from zymotic diseases; 2d, by a smaller, but still very large increase in the mortality from local diseases; 3rd, by a diminution in the mortality from constitutional diseases. We will next proceed to enquire what orders in these several classes of diseases are most concerned in bringing about these changes.

TABLE NO. 4.

Deaths of Male Citizens of the United States between the Ages of fifteen and fifty, during the Year ending June 1st, 1860, from the Several Orders of Diseases, with the Ratio of such Deaths per 1000 of Population of Corresponding Ages, and also per 1000 of Deaths from all Diseases, by Regions.

ORDERS	ATLANTIC REGION			CENTRAL REGION			PACIFIC REGION			TOTAL		
	DEATHS	Ratio per 1000 of male population between the ages of 15 and 50.	Ratio per 1000 of deaths of males between the ages of 15 and 50.	DEATHS	Ratio per 1000 of male population between the ages of 15 and 50.	Ratio per 1000 of deaths of males between the ages of 15 and 50.	DEATHS	Ratio per 1000 of male population between the ages of 15 and 50.	Ratio per 1000 of deaths of males between the ages of 15 and 50.	DEATHS	Ratio per 1000 of male population between the ages of 15 and 50.	Ratio per 1000 of deaths of males between the ages of 15 and 50.
I. 1. Miasmatic Diseases,	5,135	1.22	196.37	6,770	.50	288.20	214	.71	180.29	12,119	1.60	237.81
2. Enthetic Diseases,	27	.007	1.03	35	.01	1.49	22	.07	18.53	84	.01	1.65
3. Dietic Diseases,	518	.12	19.71	406	.11	17.24	35	.12	29.48	958	.12	18.80
II. 1. Diathetic Diseases,	1,463	.33	63.38	1,132	.32	48.19	82	.28	69.08	2,617	.33	51.36
2. Tubercular Diseases,	9,174	2.18	349.04	6,532	1.55	276.49	344	1.14	281.81	16,050	1.87	295.32
III. 1. Parasitic Diseases,	6	.001	.23	6	.001	.96	2	.007	1.69	14	.002	.28
IV. 1. Diseases of the Nervous System	2,207	.55	83.57	1,816	.51	77.27	96	.32	80.88	4,118	.51	80.81
4. Diseases of Organs of Circulat'n	827	.20	31.47	335	.09	14.26	61	.20	51.38	1,223	.16	24.00
5. Diseases of Respiratory Organs,	2,796	.77	106.33	4,080	1.16	173.68	87	.29	62.34	6,949	.86	136.36
6. Diseases of Digestive Organs,	1,470	.35	55.93	1,297	.36	55.21	74	.25	63.30	2,854	.36	66.00
7. Dis. of Urinary and Genital Orgs	203	.06	10.00	174	.06	7.41	14	.05	11.80	451	.06	8.85
8. Diseases of Bones and Joints,	32	.008	1.22	40	.01	1.70	4	.01	3.37	76	.01	1.49
9. Diseases of Integumentary Sys.	150	.04	5.71	111	.03	4.73	16	.05	13.18	277	.04	5.43
VI. Unclassified,	2,276	.51	86.60	1,759	.49	74.88	136	.45	114.67	4,171	.52	81.84
Total,	26,283	6.26	1000.00	23,491	0.58	1000.00	1,167	3.95	1000.00	50,961	6.31	1000.00

TABLE NO. 5.

Deaths in the Armies of the United States during the Year ending June 30th, 1862, from the Several Orders of Diseases, with the Ratio of such Deaths per 1000 of Mean Strength, and also per 1000 of Deaths from all Diseases, by Regions.

ORDERS	ATLANTIC REGION			CENTRAL REGION			PACIFIC REGION			TOTAL		
	DEATHS	Ratio per 1000 of mean strength	Ratio per 1000 of deaths from all diseases	DEATHS	Ratio per 1000 of mean strength	Ratio per 1000 of deaths from all diseases	DEATHS	Ratio per 1000 of men strength	Ratio per 1000 of deaths from all diseases	DEATHS	Ratio per 1000 of mean strength	Ratio per 1000 of deaths from all diseases
I. 1. Miasmatic Diseases,	3,989	21.85	669.97	5,216	51.11	639.84	30	4.48	389.61	9,235	31.74	651.13
2. Enthetic Diseases,	5	.02	.84	8	.08	.98				13	.04	.92
II. 1. Dietic Diseases,	38	.21	6.38	45	.44	5.52	2	.30	25.97	85	.30	5.99
2. Diathetic Diseases,	38	.21	6.38	62	.61	7.61	6	.89	77.92	106	.36	7.48
III. Tubercular Diseases,	247	1.35	41.49	305	3.00	37.41	8	1.19	103.90	560	1.92	39.48
IV. Parasitic Diseases,												
V. 1. Diseases of Nervous System,	232	1.27	38.97	233	2.29	28.58	9	1.34	116.88	474	1.63	33.42
2. Diseases of the Eye,				1	.01	.12				1	.003	.07
3. Diseases of the Ear,				4	.04	.49				4	.01	.28
4. Diseases of Organs of Circulat'n.	68	.37	11.42	61	.60	7.49	4	.60	51.95	133	.46	9.38
5. Diseases of Respiratory Organs,	866	4.74	145.45	1,797	17.67	220.44	8	1.19	103.90	2,671	9.18	188.33
6. Diseases of Digestive Organs,	183	1.00	30.74	225	2.21	27.60	5	.75	64.94	413	1.42	29.12
7. Dis. of Urinary and Genital Orgs	22	.12	3.69	8	.08	.98				30	.10	2.11
8. Diseases of Bones and Joints,				1	.01	.12				1	.003	.07
9. Diseases of Integumentary Sys.	4	.02	.67	11	.11	1.35				15	.05	1.06
VI. Unclassified,	262	1.43	44.00	175	1.72	21.47	5	.75	64.94	442	1.52	31.16
Total,	5,954	32.59	1000.00	8,152	80.18	1000.00	77	11.49	1000.00	14,183	48.74	1000.00

TABLE NO. 6.

Deaths in the Armies of the United States during the Year ending June 30th, 1863, from the Several Orders of Diseases, with the Ratio of such Deaths per 1000 of Mean Strength, and also per 1000 of Deaths from all Diseases, by Regions.

ORDERS.	ATLANTIC REGION.			CENTRAL REGION.			PACIFIC REGION.			TOTAL.		
	DEATHS.	Ratio per 1000 of mean strength.	Ratio per 1000 of deaths from all diseases.	DEATHS.	Ratio per 1000 of mean strength.	Ratio per 1000 of deaths from all diseases.	DEATHS.	Ratio per 1000 of mean strength.	Ratio per 1000 of deaths from all diseases.	DEATHS.	Ratio per 1000 of mean strength.	Ratio per 1000 of deaths from all diseases.
I. 1. Miasmatic Diseases	9395	30.16	729.57	19903	61.57	667.60	17	1.95	232.88	29380	45.58	699.36
2. Enthetic Diseases	13	.04	1.01	20	.19	1.00	4	.45	54.79	46	.07	1.09
II. 1. Dietic Diseases	121	.39	9.39	161	.33	5.55	2	.23	27.40	284	.44	6.76
2. Diathetic Diseases	167	.54	12.95	301	.93	10.37				463	.73	11.14
Tubercular Diseases	645	2.07	50.01	1335	4.43	49.41	8	.92	109.59	2083	3.24	49.71
III. Parasitic Diseases	1	.003	.08							1	.002	.02
IV. 1. Diseases of Nervous System	567	1.82	43.96	917	2.83	31.58	7	.90	95.89	1491	2.31	35.50
2. Diseases of the Eye	2	.006	.16		.003	.03				3	.006	.07
3. Diseases of the Ear												
4. Disease of Organs of Circulat'n	286	.85	20.63	320	.99	11.02	5	.57	63.49	591	.92	14.07
5. Diseases of Respiratory Organs	1188	3.81	92.17	4818	14.85	166.94	13	1.49	178.05	6019	9.34	143.25
6. Diseases of Digestive Organs	445	1.43	34.50	914	2.82	31.47	15	1.72	205.49	1374	2.13	32.70
7. Dis. Urinary and Genital Orgs	63	.20	4.89	53	.29	3.20	2	.25	27.40	158	.25	3.76
8. Diseases of Bones and Joints	4	.01	.31	25	.08	.86				29	.05	.69
9. Dis. of Integumentary System	20	.06	1.55	59	.18	2.00				79	.12	1.86
Total	12397	41.39	1000.00	23040	99.56	1000.00	73	8.27	100.00	43910	65.19	1000.00

We see from these tables that in the production of the greatly increased mortality by zymotic diseases in our armies, as compared with that produced by the same class of diseases in civil life, the order *miasmatic* was chiefly concerned. Of the local diseases the four most important orders arranged in the order of their relative fatality, in men of military ages in civil life, are: 1st, diseases of the respiratory organs; 2d, diseases of the nervous system; 3d, diseases of the digestive organs; and, 4th, diseases of the organs of circulation. Of these, the diseases of the respiratory organs are much the most important, producing almost as great a total mortality as the other three orders combined. We find, moreover, by comparing the ratios of deaths from each of these orders of diseases per 1000 of living in civil life, and in our armies, that diseases of the respiratory organs were chiefly concerned in producing that increase of mortality from local diseases, which, as we have already shown, existed in our armies. Thus we find that in civil life the reported deaths from diseases of the respiratory organs amounted to less than one per 1000 of living, while in our armies it amounted to nine and one-fourth per 1000 of mean strength. The mortality from diseases of the respiratory organs in our armies, therefore, was very nearly eleven times as great as that reported in civil life, while that from diseases of the nervous system was but little over three times as great during the first year, and somewhat less than five times as great during the second year of the war; that from diseases of the digestive organs four times as great during the first year, and six times as great during the second year; and that from diseases of the organs of circulation three times as great during the first year, and six times as great during the second year, as that produced by the same orders respectively in civil life. The total mortality from disease in our armies was: for the first year nearly eight times, and for the second year ten times as great as that reported in civil life. The proportional increase of mortality from diseases of the respiratory organs, therefore, was considerably above the average, while that from the other three orders named was far below such average. The mortality from all these orders was, however, evidently increased somewhat, especially during the second year of the war. We find, then, that the increase of mortality in our armies over that which occurs in men of military ages in civil life, was confined chiefly, though not exclusively, to two orders of diseases, namely : *the miasmatic diseases, and diseases of the respiratory organs.* In respect to the diseases of the respiratory organs, it is not necessary to our present purpose to pursue our inquiries farther; nor if it were, would the nature of our statistics make the conclusions to which we might arrive, worthy of confidence. In the order of diseases named, *miasmatic,* on the contrary, are included diseases, so different in their nature and general appearance, that the order may be divided into several groups, separated from each other by such well marked lines of division as render them little liable to be confounded. Such division of this order is the more necessary from the fact that the individual diseases of which it is composed, are produced by different causes, and point to different hygienic means for their prevention.

For the purpose of comparison, therefore, I shall divide the order miasmatic into four groups, namely : 1st, fevers; 2d, diarrhœa and dysentery; 3d, intermittents; and, 4th, the infectious diseases, the most important representatives of which, in our army, were small-pox and measles. I am aware that so far as causation is concerned, these groups are not all separated by well marked lines. The intermittents, for example, do not represent the whole of the action of malaria. Undoubtedly many fevers reported as typhoid, typho-malarial and remittent, were chiefly or wholly caused by malaria; but there is good reason to believe that many others reported under these heads were entirely independent of any malarial influence. While grouping remittent and typho-malarial fevers with the fevers, therefore, it is to be born in mind that some of these diseases were undoubtedly of malarial origin, while others were produced by entirely different causes. Again, typhoid fever, the most fatal disease in our armies, if accuracy of diagnosis could be relied upon, should, in my opinion, be classed with small-pox and measles, as belonging to the family of diseases produced by the specific disease poisons. But how far the cases reported as typhoid fever were produced by the typhoid fever poison, and how far they were produced by malaria and other causes, it is impossible exactly to determine.

TABLE NO. 7.

Annual Mortality in the Armies of the United States, and in Male Citizens of the United States between the ages of fifteen and fifty, from Fevers, expressed in Ratio per 1000 of Mean Strength, and also in Ratio per 1000 of total Annual Deaths from all Diseases.

| | ARMIES OF THE UNITED STATES. | | | | | | MALE CITIZENS OF THE U.S. BETWEEN THE AGES OF 15 AND 50. | | |
| | YEAR ENDING JUNE 30, 1862. | | | YEAR ENDING JUNE 30, 1863. | | | YEAR ENDING JUNE 1, 1860. | | |
	DEATHS.	Ratio per 1000 of mean strength.	Ratio per 1000 of deaths from all diseases.	DEATHS.	Ratio per 1000 of mean strength.	Ratio per 1000 of deaths from all diseases.	DEATHS.	Ratio per 1000 of male population between 15 and 50.	Ratio per 1000 of deaths between the ages of 15 to 50 from all diseases.
Typhus Fever,	191	.66	13.47	381	.50	9.07			
Typhoid Fever,	5,608	19.28	395.40	10,467	16.24	249.15	6,099	.76	119.68
Typho-Malarial Fever,				1,129	1.75	26.87			
Common Continued Fever,	146	.50	10.29						
Remittent Fever,	370	1.27	26.09	1,167	1.81	27.78	2,007	.25	39.38
Total,	6,315	21.71	445.25	13,144	20.39	312.87	8,106	1.01	159.06

TABLE NO. 8.

Annual Mortality in the Armies of the United States, and in Male Citizens of the United States, between the ages of fifteen and fifty, from Diarrhœa and Dysentery, expressed in Ratio per 1000 of Mean Strength, and also in Ratio per 1000 of Total Annual Deaths from all Diseases.

	ARMIES OF THE UNITED STATES.						MALE CITIZENS OF THE U. S. BETWEEN THE AGES OF 15 AND 50.		
	YEAR ENDING JUNE 30, 1862.			YEAR ENDING JUNE 30, 1863.			YEAR ENDING JUNE 1, 1860.		
	DEATHS.	Ratio per 1000 of mean strength.	Ratio per 1000 of deaths from all diseases.	DEATHS.	Ratio per 1000 of mean strength.	Ratio per 1000 of deaths from all diseases.	DEATHS.	Ratio per 1000 of male population between the ages of 15 and 50.	Ratio per 1000 of deaths of males between the ages of 15 and 50, from all diseases.
Acute Diarrhœa,	227	.78	16.00	870	1.35	20.71	544	.07	10.67
Chronic Diarrhœa,	193	1.69	34.76	7,488	11.62	178.34			
Acute Dysentery,	317	1.19	21.47	922	1.43	21.95	828	.10	16.25
Chronic Dysentery,	127	.44	8.95	1,086	1.68	25.85			
Total,	1194	4.10	84.18	10,366	16.08	246.75	1,372	.17	26.92

TABLE NO. 9.

Annual Mortality in the Armies of the United States, and in Male Citizens of the United States, between the ages of fifteen and fifty, from Intermittents, expressed in Ratio per 1000 of Mean Strength, and also in Ratio per 1000 of Total Annual Deaths from all Diseases.

| | ARMIES OF THE UNITED STATES. | | | | | | MALE CITIZENS OF THE U. S. BETWEEN THE AGES OF 15 AND 50. | | |
| | YEAR ENDING JUNE 30, 1862. | | | YEAR ENDING JUNE 30, 1863. | | | YEAR ENDING JUNE 1, 1860. | | |
	DEATHS.	Ratio per 1000 of mean strength.	Ratio per 1000 of deaths from all diseases.	DEATHS.	Ratio per 1000 of mean strength.	Ratio per 1000 of deaths from all diseases.	DEATHS.	Ratio per 1000 of male population between the ages of 15 and 50.	Ratio per 1000 of deaths of males between the ages of 15 and 50, from all diseases.
Quotidian Intermittents,	32	.11	2.26	144	.22	3.43			
Tertian Intermittents,	33	.11	2.33	116	.18	2.76			
Quartan Intermittents,	4	.01	.28	78	.12	1.86			
Congestive Intermittents,	361	1.24	25.45	1,020	1.58	24.28	762	.09	14.95
Total,	430	1.48	30.32	1,358	2.11	32.33	762	.09	14.95

TABLE NO. 10.

Annual Mortality in the Armies of the United States, and in Male Citizens of the United States, between the ages of fifteen and fifty, from Small Pox and Measles, expressed in Ratio per 1000 of Mean Strength, and also in Ratio per 1000 of Total Annual Deaths from all Diseases.

	ARMIES OF THE UNITED STATES.					MALE CITIZENS OF THE U. S. BETWEEN THE AGES OF 15 AND 50.		
	YEAR ENDING JUNE 30, 1862.			YEAR ENDING JUNE 30, 1863.			YEAR ENDING JUNE 1, 1860.		
	DEATHS.	Ratio per 1000 of mean strength.	Ratio per 1000 of deaths from all diseases.	DEATHS.	Ratio per 1000 of mean strength.	Ratio per 1000 of deaths from all diseases.	DEATHS.	Ratio per 1000 of Male population betwen the ages of 15 and 50.	Ratio per 1000 of deaths of males between the ages of 15 and 50, from all diseases.
Small Pox and Varioloid,............	412	1.42	29.05	1,132	1.76	26.95	295	.04	5.79
Measles,.......................	551	1.89	38.85	1,313	2.04	31.25	190	.02	3.73
Total,............................	963	3.31	67.90	2,445	3.80	58.20	485	.06	9.52

We see from Table No. 7, that while the family of fevers caused but 160 of every 1000 deaths in men of military ages in civil life, in our armies it caused during the first year of the war 445, and during the second year 313 of every 1000 deaths; and we find, upon farther examination, that the smaller proportional mortality during the second year is almost wholly owing to a relative increase in the mortality from other diseases. The ratio per 1000 of Mean Strength was indeed but little less during the second year than during the first.

Diarrhœa and Dysentery constitute the second group in importance. We see from Table No. 8, that while these diseases caused but 27 of every 1000 deaths reported in civil life, in our armies during the first year they caused 84, and during the second year 247 of every 1000 deaths from disease. If we compare the ratio per 1000 of living, we find that during the first year of the war it was twenty-four times as great as that of the reported deaths in civil life, and that this was almost quadrupled during the second year.

From Table No. 9, we see that, while Intermittents caused but 15 of every 1000 deaths in civil life, they caused in our armies from 30 to 32 of every 1000 deaths. Although the mortality from these diseases was comparatively small, they were clearly much more prevalent and fatal in our armies than in civil life.

From Table No. 10, we see that, while Small Pox and Measles, together caused but 10 of every 1000 reported deaths in civil life, in our armies they caused 68 per 1000 of deaths during the first year, and 58 per 1000 during the second year; and that the ratio of deaths from these diseases per 1000 of living became increased from .06 per 1000 in civil life to 33 per 1000 during the first year of the war, and 38 per 1000 during the second year.

The following table will, perhaps, exhibit more clearly the relative influence which these several groups of diseases exerted upon the mortality of our armies during the first two years of the war :

TABLE NO. 11.

Annual Mortality in the Armies of the United States, and in Male Citizens of the United States, between the ages of fifteen and fifty, from the several Groups of Diseases comprising the Order Miasmatic, and from diseases of the Respiratory Organs, expressed in ratio per 1000 of Mean Strength, and also in ratio per 1000 of total annual deaths from all diseases.

	ARMIES OF THE UNITED STATES.				MALE CITIZENS OF THE U. S. BETWEEN THE AGES OF 15 AND 50.	
	YEAR ENDING JUNE 30, 1862.		YEAR ENDING JUNE 30, 1863.		YEAR ENDING JUNE 1, 1860.	
	Ratio per 1000 of mean strength.	Ratio per 1000 of deaths from all diseases.	Ratio per 1000 of mean strength.	Ratio per 1000 of deaths from all diseases.	Ratio per 1000 of male population between the ages of 15 and 50.	Ratio per 1000 of deaths of males between the ages of 15 and 50, from all diseases.
Fevers,	21.71	445.25	20.39	312.87	1.01	159.06
Diarrhœa and Dysentery,	4.10	81.18	16.08	246.75	.17	28.92
Intermittents,	1.48	30.32	2.11	32.33	.09	14.96
Small Pox and Measles,	3.51	67.90	3.80	58.20	.06	9.52
Diseases of the Respiratory Organs,	9.18	188.33	9.34	143.28	.86	136.36
All other Diseases,	8.97	184.02	13.47	206.57	4.13	653.19
Total,	48.75	1000.00	65.19	1000.00	6.32	1000.00

4

If we compare the ratios of deaths from any one of these groups of diseases per 1000 of deaths from all diseases in civil life, and in our armies during either year, we find that all the groups named represent a mortality terribly excessive in our armies, while the deaths from all other diseases are, for the first year but 184, and for the second year 207 of every 1000 deaths in our armies, against 653 of every 1000 in civil life. The most striking increase in mortality during the second year of the war over that of the first year, was produced by diarrhœa and dysentery. These diseases caused but 84 deaths of every 1000 during the first year, and 247 during the second year; almost three times as large a proportion. A comparison of the ratios of deaths to living gives similar results, and is equally instructive. By reason of the probable incompleteness of the mortality statistics of civil life, it cannot be assumed that the ratios of deaths per 1000 of male population between fifteen and fifty, as given in the above table, represent the actual mortality from these diseases in men of military ages in civil life. But, if we assume that the deaths not reported would be divided between the several diseases in about the same proportions as those reported; and that, upon the whole, one half of all the deaths was reported; then, by multiplying the ratios in the table by two, they will be made to represent the true ratios of the actual mortality. Doubling the ratios of deaths per 1000 of living in civil life, and comparing them with the ratios of deaths from corresponding groups of diseases per 1000 of Mean Strength in our armies, we find that the mortality from fevers was approximately ten times as great in our armies as in men of military ages in civil life; that from diarrhœa and dysentery during the first year of the war, twenty-three times as great, and during the second year, eighty-nine times as great; that from intermittents about twelve times as great during the first year, and eighteen times as great during the second year; that from small pox and measles about ten times as great; and that from diseases of the respiratory organs something over five times as great; while that from all other diseases is about the same as in civil life during the first year, and about one and one-half times as great during the second year. It is certain, therefore, that the five groups of diseases above named were chiefly instrumental in producing the excess of mortality which occurred in our armies over that which occurs in men of military ages in civil life; and that arranged in the order of their importance they would stand for the first year of the war: first, fevers; second, diseases of the respiratory organs; third, diarrhœa and dysentery; fourth, small pox and measles; and fifth, intermittents. But for the second year: first, fevers; second, diarrhœa and dysentery; third, diseases of the respiratory organs; &c.

It remains now to inquire respecting the relative mortality from these several groups of diseases in the different regions:

TABLE NO. 12.

Deaths of Male Citizens of the United States between the Ages of fifteen and fifty, during the Year ending June 1st, 1860, from the Several Groups of Diseases embraced in the Order Miasmatic, and from Diseases of the Respiratory Organs, with the Ratio per 1000 of Male Population of Corresponding Ages, and also the Ratio per 1000 of Deaths from all Diseases, by Regions.

	ATLANTIC REGION.			CENTRAL REGION.			PACIFIC REGION.			TOTAL.		
	DEATHS.	Ratio per 1000 of male population between the ages of 15 and 50.	Ratio per 1000 of deaths of males between the ages of 15 and 50, from all diseases.	DEATHS.	Ratio per 1000 of male population between the ages of 15 and 50.	Ratio per 1000 of deaths of males between the ages of 15 and 50, from all diseases.	DEATHS.	Ratio per 1000 of male population between the ages of 15 and 50.	Ratio per 1000 of deaths of males between the ages of 15 and 50.	DEATHS.	Ratio per 1000 of male population between the ages of 15 and 50.	Ratio per 1000 of deaths of males between the ages of 15 and 50, from all diseases.
Fevers,..........	3,656	.87	139.10	4,330	1.21	184.33	120	.39	101.10	8,106	1.01	159.06
Diarrhœa and Dysentery,....	486	.12	18.49	845	.24	35.97	41	.14	34.54	1,372	.17	26.92
Intermittents,....	146	.03	5.56	586	.16	24.95	30	.10	25.28	762	.09	14.95
Small Pox and Measles,......	327	.08	12.44	153	.04	6.51	5	.02	4.21	485	.06	9.52
Diseases of Respiratory Organs,....	2,795	.67	106.34	4,080	1.15	173.68	74	.25	62.34	6,949	.86	136.36
All other Diseases,.......	18,873	4.50	718.07	13,497	3.78	574.56	917	3.05	772.53	33,287	4.13	653.19
Total,......	26,283	6.26	1000.00	23,491	6.58	1000.00	1,187	3 95	1000.00	50,961	6.32	1000.00

TABLE NO. 13.

Deaths in the Armies of the United States during the Year ending June 30th, 1862, from the Several Groups of Diseases embraced in the Order Miasmatic, and from Diseases of the Respiratory Organs, with the Ratio per 1000 of Mean Strength, and also the Ratio per 1000 of Deaths from all Diseases, by Regions.

	ATLANTIC REGION.			CENTRAL REGION.			PACIFIC REGION.			TOTAL.		
	DEATHS.	Ratio per 1000 of mean strength.	Ratio per 1000 of deaths from all diseases.	DEATHS.	Ratio per 1000 of mean strength.	Ratio per 1000 of deaths from all diseases.	DEATHS.	Ratio per 1000 of mean strength.	Ratio per 1000 of deaths from all diseases.	DEATHS.	Ratio per 1000 of mean strength.	Ratio per 1000 of deaths from all diseases.
Fevers, ...	3,059	16.75	513.77	3,245	31.92	398.06	11	1.64	142.86	6,315	21.71	445.25
Diarrhœa and Dysentery, ...	238	1.30	39.97	951	9.36	116.66	5	.75	64.93	1,194	4.10	84.18
Intermittents, ...	210	1.15	35.27	220	2.16	26.99	......	......	......	430	1.48	30.32
Small Pox and Measles, ...	383	2.10	64.33	567	5.58	69.55	13	1.94	168.83	963	3.31	67.90
Diseases of Respiratory Organs,..	866	4.74	145.45	1,797	17.67	220.44	8	1.19	103.90	2,671	9.18	188.33
All other Diseases,....................	1,198	6.56	201.21	1,372	13.50	168.30	40	5.95	519.48	2,610	8.97	184.02
Total, ...	5,954	32.60	1000.00	8,152	80.19	1000.00	77	11.47	1000.00	14,183	48.75	1000.00

TABLE NO. 14.

Deaths in the Armies of the United States during the Year ending June 30th, 1863, from the Several Groups of Diseases embraced in the Order Miasmatic, and from Diseases of the Respiratory Organs, with the Ratio per 1000 of Mean Strength, and also the Ratio per 1000 of Deaths from all Diseases, by Regions.

	ATLANTIC REGION.			CENTRAL REGION.			PACIFIC REGION.			TOTAL.		
	DEATHS.	Ratio per 1000 of mean strength.	Ratio per 1000 of deaths from all diseases.	DEATHS.	Ratio per 1000 of mean strength.	Ratio per 1000 of deaths from all diseases.	DEATHS.	Ratio per 1000 of mean strength.	Ratio per 1000 of deaths from all diseases.	DEATHS.	Ratio per 1000 of mean strength.	Ratio per 1000 of deaths from all diseases.
Fevers,	5,312	17.05	411.88	7,826	24.13	269.49	6	.69	82.19	13,144	20.39	312.87
Diarrhœa and Dysentery,	2,742	8.80	212.60	7,617	23.49	262.29	7	.80	95.89	10,366	16.08	246.75
Intermittents,	297	.95	23.03	1,060	3.27	36.50	1	.11	13.70	1,358	2.11	32.33
Small Pox and Measles,	485	1.55	37.61	1,960	6.04	67.50				2,445	3.80	58.20
Diseases of Respiratory Organs,	1,188	3.81	92.12	4,818	14.85	165.91	13	1.49	178.08	6,019	9.34	143.28
All other Diseases,	2,873	9.22	222.76	5,759	17.76	198.31	46	5.28	630.14	8,678	13.47	206.57
Total,	12,897	41.40	1000.00	29,040	89.55	1000.00	73	8.37	1000.00	42,010	65.19	1000.00

Table No. 12 shows that in civil life fevers are the most fatal in the Central Region, and the least so in the Pacific Region; that the intermittents produce five times as great mortality in the Central Region as in the Atlantic; and that in the Pacific Region the proportional mortality from these diseases is as great as in the Central Region, and the ratio per 1000 of living about two-thirds as great. The mortality from diarrhœa and dysentery seems to be about twice as great in the Central Region as in the Atlantic, and in the Pacific Region the mortality seems to range between these two. Small pox and measles produced twice as great mortality in the Atlantic Region as in the Central, and least of all in the Pacific; but this was probably less dependent upon climatic influences than the difference in the mortality from the other groups. The mortality from diseases of the respiratory organs was greatest in the Central Region and least in the Pacific; that from all other diseases was greatest in the Atlantic Region.

From Table No. 13, we see that during the first year of the war, the mortality from fevers was twice as great per 1000 of mean strength in the Central Region as in the Atlantic, while in the Pacific Region it was only one-tenth as great as in the Atlantic. Comparing these ratios with corresponding ratios in Table No. 12, we see that the excess of mortality from fevers in our armies over that in civil life was about one-and-a-half times as great in the Central Region as in the Atlantic, while that in the Pacific Region approximated very closely to the average in men of military ages in civil life. In the mortality from intermittents, there is less difference between the Atlantic and Central Regions than in civil life, and in the Pacific Region no deaths were reported from these diseases. The mortality from diarrhœa and dysentery, we find to have been least in the Pacific Region, and greatest in the Central; and the difference in the mortality in the Atlantic and Central Regions is very striking, being over seven times as great in the latter as in the former, while in civil life it was just twice as great. Small pox and measles were here the most fatal in the Central Region. The mortality from diseases of the respiratory organs was nearly four times as great in the Central as in the Atlantic Region, while in civil life it was less than twice as great.

During the second year the mortality from fevers remained about the same in the Atlantic Region as during the first year, while in both the Central and Pacific Regions it was decidedly less. The mortality from diarrhœa and dysentery increased in the Atlantic Region from 1.3 per 1000 of mean strength—the mortality during the first year—to 8.8 per 1000; and in the Central Region from 9.36 per 1000 of mean strength to 23.49 per 1000, while in the Pacific Region the mortality from these diseases remained about the same as during the first year of the war. The mortality from small pox and measles was about four times as great in the Central Region as in the Atlantic, while in the Pacific Region none were lost from either of these diseases. Diseases of the respiratory organs produced almost four times as much mortality in the Central Region as in the Atlantic, and ten times as much as in the Pacific Region—the relative mortality in the several regions being nearly the same as during the first year. The mortality from all other diseases was nearly twice as great in the Central Region as in the Atlantic, and somewhat more than three times as great as in the Pacific Region—the relative mortality in the several regions differing but little from that of the 1st year.

We find, therefore, that in our armies the excess of mortality over that which occurs in men of military ages in civil life, was caused almost wholly by a few groups of diseases, namely: fevers, diarrhœa and dysentery, diseases of the respiratory organs, and the infectious diseases. Was this peculiar to our armies or does it agree with the experience of the armies of other nations? In the British army in the Crimea, the annual mortality from diseases reached 232 per 1000 of mean strength, over three and a half times as great as in our armies during the second year of the war.

The following table shows what diseases were most influential in causing this great mortality.

TABLE NO. 15.

Annual Average of mortality in the British Army in the Crimea from September 1854, to June 1856, from Several Groups of Diseases, with the Ratio of such mortality per 1000 of Average Mean Strength, and also per 1000 of Annual Average of Total Deaths from all Diseases.

	Deaths.—Annual Average.	Ratio of annual deaths per 1000 of average mean strength.	Ratio of annual deaths per 1000 of annual average of total deaths from all diseases.
Fevers, (not typhus)	1,897	45.17	195.02
Diarrhœa and Dysentery,	3,546	84.58	364.55
Cholera and Typhus,	2,879	68.45	295.98
All other Diseases,	1,405	33.51	144.45
Total,	9,727	231.71	1000.00

We see from this table that over five-sixths of all the mortality from disease in the British army of the Crimea was caused by three of the same four groups of diseases that caused the chief mortality in our armies, namely: fevers; diarrhœa and dysentery; and the infectious diseases. The relative mortality from these several groups, however, is not the same as in our armies. In the British Crimean army the mortality from diarrhœa and dysentery was considerably greater than that from any other group of diseases, reaching 85 per 1000 of mean strength—a mortality considerably greater than the total mortality from disease in our armies during the second year.

Next to diarrhœa and dysentery in fatality, stand the infectious diseases, represented by two, from the ravages of which our armies were almost if not wholly exempt. The mortality from cholera and typhus amounted to 69 per 1000 of mean strength—greater than the total mortality from disease in our armies. These groups of diseases, therefore, arranged in the order of their fatality in the British Crimean army, would stand: first, diarrhœa and dysentery; second, infectious diseases; third fevers. It is to be noticed, also, that while the mortality from each of these groups was much larger than in our own army, this excess was especially marked in the diseases produced by the specific disease poisons, and in diarrhœa and dysentery. In the French army in the Crimea, the mortality was even greater than in the British army. The following table embraces only the mortality which occurred in the Crimea, not including that in the hospitals at Constantinople and other places. As many of the sick were transferred to the hospitals at Constantinople and other places, the ratio of deaths per 1000 of mean strength is not given; but the total annual mortality from disease scarcely fell short of 300 per 1000 of mean strength.

TABLE NO. 16.

Deaths in the French Army in the Crimea from September 1854 *to July* 1856, *from Several Groups of Diseases, with the Ratio of such Deaths per* 1000 *of total Deaths from all Diseases.*

	DEATHS.	Ratio per 1000 of al deaths from disease in the Crimea.
Fevers, (not typhus)	5,458	226.38
Diarrhœa and Dysentery,	4,045	167.77
Cholera and Typhus,	12,031	499.00
All other Diseases,	2,576	106.85
Total,	24,110	1000.00

We see here the relative influence of the same groups of diseases in producing the terrible mortality which the French troops suffered. One-half of all this terrible mortality was produced by two specific disease poisons, namely: cholera and typhus. The proportional mortality from fevers was also greater than in the British army, while that from diarrhœa and dysentery was less than half as great. But the three groups of diseases named caused almost nine-tenths of the total mortality from disease in the Crimea.

I think it clear, therefore, that the groups of diseases we have named, are those chiefly concerned in producing the great mortality which has ever attended all great military campaigns. Upon what circumstances connected with military life, is the excessive mortality from these several groups of diseases dependent? As has already been intimated, there was probably no one cause which alone produced any one of these diseases or groups of diseases, and which did not, at the same time, affect the mortality of other diseases. The same cause was undoubtedly often concerned in increasing the fatality of different diseases.

The greater mortality from fevers, diarrhœa and dysentery, and diseases of the respiratory organs in the Central Region than in the Atlantic or Pacific Regions was, undoubtedly, in great part due to the influence of the malarial poison. And overcrowding in camps, barracks, and hospitals; and imperfect nutrition, by deteriorating and depraving the blood and weakening the vital forces, undoubtedly contributed to the fatality of all diseases, but not to all alike. Most of these causes should undoubtedly be considered as factors in the production of the mortality from any one of these groups of diseases; so that it is by no means easy to isolate and compare the relative influence of each cause. Still, certain causes were, evidently, especially influential in the production of certain diseases, or in increasing their fatality. The most important of these causes were, I think, overcrowding in camps, barracks and hospitals; imperfect nutrition; malaria; the specific disease poisons, and exposure. And while the mortality from all diseases was probably increased by the associated action of most of these causes, several of them certainly had a more direct and marked effect upon the mortality of some diseases than of others. There is perhaps no single cause, certainly none if we except an insufficient ration, which has exerted a greater influence upon the mortality of armies than overcrowding. This has been especially destructive when any specific disease poison has been present; but its influence upon the mortality of all diseases has been very great. For one, I do not doubt, that the low rate of mortality in our armies during the late war, compared with the mortality of other large armies, was largely due to our ample and well ventilated hospitals. It may be said without fear of contradiction, that in no large military hospitals in the world was the mortality ever before so low.

The following table shows the mortality from wounds and diseases treated in the French hospitals at Constantinople during the Crimean war. The table is from the work of M. Scrive, inspector general of the French Medical Service in the Crimea, and is quoted by Dr. Macleod, in his Notes on the Surgery of the Crimean war, page 372.

TABLE NO. 17.

Table showing the Wounds and Diseases treated in the hospitals at Constantinople during the war:

	Transferred from Varna or the Crimea	Admissions at Constantinople	Dismissed, Cured, or Well.	Transferr'd	Died.
Wounds, (ordinary)	2,185	1,007	2,059	720	413
" by gunshot,	22,891	....	9,616	8,190	5,085
Frost-bite, ...	3,472	142	2,009	775	830
Typhus,..................	3,840	4,889	3,544	1,778	3,407
Cholera, ...	3,196	2,570	2,529	1,076	2,161
Scurvy,..................	17,576	3,851	9,587	8,460	3,380
Fever,...................	63,124	8,038	35,625	22,988	12,549
Venereal, ...	241	2,597	2,316	522	....
Skin affections(itch)	124	156	256	24	....
	116,649	23,250	67,541	44,533	27,825
	139,899		139,899		

Deducting those transferred from the total admissions, as cases not terminated, and we have a mortality of one death to every three patients, almost : or nearly 33 per cent.; whereas in our own hospitals, Dr. Woodward* says, " Making proper corrections for transfers from hospital to hospital, there were over a million of patients treated in the general hospitals during the four years of the war, and the mortality, including both that from disease and that from wounds, was but one death to every twelve patients, or about eight per cent."

It was not until during the second year of the war that ridge ventilated hospitals were provided to any considerable extent; and it is worthy of notice in this connection, that while the mortality from all the other groups of diseases underwent a more or less marked increase during the second year of the war, the mortality from fevers diminished. There is small reason to doubt that this diminution was chiefly due to the more ample and better ventilated hospitals provided during the second year, for I believe no other cause of disease underwent any diminution in intensity. The remarkably low mortality in our immense

*Circular No. 6, Surgeon General's Office, p. 158.

military hospitals as compared with other large military hospitals, is, undoubtedly, chiefly attributable to the same cause. It
is, therefore, undoubtedly true, that our excellent system of hospitals rendered the mortality from all diseases and from wounds
much less than it would have been under other circumstances;
but that the mortality from fevers was diminished in a more
marked degree than that from any other group of diseases. But
notwithstanding the restraining influence which our better hospital accommodations undoubtedly exerted upon the mortality
of the second year of the war, we find that the mortality from
diarrhœa and dysentery leaped from 4.1 per 1000 of mean
strength during the first year, to 16.08 per 1000 during the
second year—a mortality four-fifths as great as that from fevers.
This was certainly the most remarkable phenomenon in the
mortality of the second year of the war, and is deserving of
careful consideration. It is probably true that no single cause
was alone concerned in the causation of these diseases. But, I
think, the conclusion is irresistible that some cause was here at
work, and one, too, of great power and effect, which exerted an
influence upon the fatality of these diseases, vastly greater than
it exerted upon the fatality of any other group of diseases whatever. What was this cause? It is, I think, undeniable, as
claimed by Dr. Woodward, that both heat and malaria were
active auxiliary causes in the production of these diseases; but
it is, I think, equally undeniable that the remarkable increase
of mortality from these diseases during the second year of the
war cannot be rationally attributed, chiefly, or even to any important extent, to either, or both of these causes. That malaria
had comparatively little to do with this increase is, I think, clear,
from two facts: first, the mortality from intermittents underwent
no such great increase; the increase in the mortality from intermittents was, indeed, but little greater than the average
increase of mortality from all diseases. Second, in the Central
Region—the favorite habitat of malaria—the increase of mortality from diarrhœa and dysentery during the second year was
but little over one-third as great as in the Atlantic Region; the
relation of the mortality from these diseases during the first and
second years of the war respectively, being, in the Atlantic Re-

gion as 1.3 to 8.8, and in the Central Region as 9.36 to 23.49.
Nor was the latitude in which the troops served during the second year so greatly different from that in which they served
during the first year, as to account, to any considerable extent,
for the remarkable increase of mortality from diarrhœa and dysentery during the second year. However great, then, the influence which these two causes exerted upon the fatality of these
diseases, and that such influence was great is, I think, beyond
question, the facts in the case do not indicate that such influence
was essentially greater during the second year of the war than
during the first year. The cause of this increase must then be
sought for elsewhere. And, I think, the facts point with a con-
clusiveness scarcely short of certainty, to some essential defi-
ciency in the ration, as the chief cause of this increase.

"The influence of the scorbutic taint," says Dr. Woodward,*
in the production of diarrhœa and dysentery is shown not only
in the increased frequency of these disorders whenever supplies
of fresh meat and vegetables have been deficient, but also by
the presence of readily recognized scorbutic symptoms in the
patients. When on marches or active campaigns, the diet is
reduced to a minimum, often consisting chiefly of hard bread and
coffee, with but a scanty supply of salt pork, and of beef on the
hoof, the number of acute attacks of a mild form, as also of
attacks which become chronic, is always increased." The relation of diarrhœa and dysentery to insufficient nutrition was shown
in the history of the British Crimean army by the great diminution in these diseases which followed the improved character of
the ration during the latter portion of the war, when Dr. Macleod says, "Every luxury prevailed in our hospitals, and our
army lived as I suppose no army has ever fared in the annals
of warfare." The insufficiency of the diet of the British soldier
during the early part of the Crimean war was much greater than
any where known in our own army at any time during the rebellion. Dr. Macleod says, "The food provided for the army
during the first winter and spring was defective both in quantity
and quality. * * * * Salt meat and biscuit constituted
the bulk of the distribution, while rice, coffee and sugar were

*Circular No. 6, Surgeon General's Office, p. 121.

occasionally but sparingly added." The results of this insufficiency of nutriment upon the sanitary condition of the Crimean
soldier was sufficiently evident. Dr. Tholozan tells us that 700
or 800 out of a total of 1,200 cases which fell under his observation in the Pera hospitals during the winter of 1854–5 had
suffered from diarrhœa or dysentery at the outset of their several ailments. "Very few indeed," says Dr. Macleod, "who
served in the Crimea throughout the first winter, escaped an
attack of dysentery: and it is in keeping with my observation
that most of those who escaped entirely were officers who seldom
ate the salt pork, but who subsisted on fresh food which their
private means enabled them to procure." But, "from April
1855 to June 1856, comparatively few cases of dysentery ap-
peared, showing how greatly the improved hygienic condition of
the army influenced the development of this 'camp pest.' "

These facts become doubly instructive when compared with
the experience of our own army in the late rebellion, in which
the mortality from these diseases during the second year of the
war, when the influence of "camp diet" had been longer in action,
and when the greater magnitude and length of the campaigns
involved further restrictions of the ration, was four times as
great as during the first year. It is also certain that imperfect
nutrition plays an important part in increasing the mortality
from other diseases and from wounds.

The facts and statistics I have cited, I think, warrant the following conclusions, namely: That the most efficient causes of
disease and death in armies within the reach of hygienic meas-
ures are, first, An insufficient supply in the ration of one or
more of the proximate principles essential to perfect nutrition ;
second, The associated influences which spring from overcrowding: and third, The specific disease poisons. The relative importance of the two last respectively, in the causation of some
of the most important diseases from which armies suffer, cannot
be considered as settled. It is certain, however, that each is
the natural ally of the other, and that their combined action has
often caused terrible destruction of life in armies. The specific
disease poisons certainly played a much more important part in
the causation of disease and death in both the British and
French Crimean armies than in our own.

www.ingramcontent.com/pod-product-compliance
Lightning Source LLC
Chambersburg PA
CBHW021600270326
41931CB00009B/1312